EMBRACING THE ORNISH LIFESTYLE

A HOLISTIC A PPROACH TO HEALTH AND WELLNESS

A.D RAMS

Contents

CHAPTER ONE

INTRODUCTION

Dr. Dean Ornish created the Ornish program, a holistic lifestyle approach that uses social support, exercise, stress reduction, and nutrition to prevent and reverse chronic diseases. Comprehensive lifestyle modifications can not only prevent but also cure heart disease and other chronic illnesses, as shown by Dr. Ornish's ground-breaking research.

The foundation of the Ornish program is the idea that lifestyle changes can significantly reduce the risk and reverse the effects of many chronic illnesses, such as obesity, type 2 diabetes, heart disease, and hypertension. Through a comprehensive approach to wellness and health, the Ornish program enables people to take charge of their health and enhance their quality of life.

We will examine the fundamental ideas, elements, and empirical data pertaining to the Ornish program's efficacy in fostering health and wellbeing in this overview. Whether you want to manage your current health concerns, avoid chronic disease, or just live a healthier lifestyle, the Ornish program provides insightful information and doable tactics to help you reach your objectives.

Dr. Dean Ornish created the comprehensive lifestyle intervention known as the Ornish Program for Reversing Heart Disease, which aims to prevent and reverse heart disease as well as other chronic illnesses. It is founded on decades of research showing that major dietary, physical activity, stress-reduction, and social support modifications can enhance cardiovascular health and general well-being.

The curriculum focuses on what are known as the "four pillars" of the Ornish lifestyle, which are four essential elements:

Healthy Eating: The Ornish approach advocates for a plant-based, whole-food diet that is minimal in processed foods, fats, and refined carbs. The focus is on reducing intake of animal products, added sugars, and harmful fats while increasing consumption of a range of fruits, vegetables, whole grains, legumes, and plant-based proteins. The diet's rich fiber, vitamin, mineral, and antioxidant content can help lower cholesterol, improve heart health, and reduce inflammation.

Frequent Exercise: The Ornish program places a strong emphasis on regular aerobic, strength, and flexibility training. Physical activity is an integral aspect of the program. The program encourages participants to do moderate-intensity aerobic activity, including brisk walking or cycling, for at least half an hour most days of the week. To increase muscle strength and endurance, strength training activities like lifting weights or utilizing resistance bands are advised to be done at least twice a week.

Stress Management: An essential part of the Ornish regimen is stress reduction, which includes practices like yoga, mindfulness, meditation, and deep breathing exercises. By lowering stress, worry, and negative emotions, these techniques assist people in improving their mental and physical health. As part of the program, participants learn and routinely practice stress management techniques to help them develop a sense of peace and relaxation in their daily life.

Social Support: Since studies have linked strong social relationships to improved health outcomes and longer lifespans, social support and connection are essential components of the Ornish program. Building and sustaining supportive relationships with family, friends, and community members is encouraged by the curriculum. Online forums, instructional courses, and group support sessions are frequently offered to encourage a sense of accountability and connection among members.

All things considered, the Ornish program provides a comprehensive approach to health and wellness that tackles the root causes of chronic illness and gives people the tools they need to adopt sustainable lifestyle adjustments. Those who follow a whole-foods, plant-based diet, exercise frequently, learn stress-reduction strategies, and build supportive social networks can lower their risk of developing chronic illnesses, improve their cardiovascular health, and generally improve their quality of life.

The history of Dr. Dean Ornish and his contributions

Renowned author, researcher, and physician Dr. Dean Ornish has devoted his professional life to examining the effects of lifestyle modifications on health and wellness, with a focus on the prevention and treatment of chronic conditions like heart disease.

Dr. Ornish was born in Dallas, Texas, on July 16, 1953, and earned a Bachelor of Arts in Humanities from the University of Texas in Austin. After that, he continued his education at Baylor College of Medicine, where he graduated with an MD. At Harvard Medical School-affiliated Massachusetts General Hospital and Beth Israel Hospital in Boston, Dr. Ornish finished his residency in medicine.

Early in his medical practice, Dr. Ornish developed an interest in lifestyle treatments and preventive medicine. He carried out ground-breaking research on the relationship between heart disease and alterations in nutrition, exercise, stress reduction, and social support in the late 1970s. His research disproved accepted knowledge by showing that significant lifestyle modifications, devoid of medication or surgery, might not only prevent but also cure cardiac disease.

In order to carry out additional research on the impact of lifestyle changes on health and disease, Dr. Ornish established the nonprofit Preventive Medicine Research Institute (PMRI) in Sausalito, California, in 1984. The institute teaches the public and medical professionals, carries out clinical research, and promotes the wider use of lifestyle-based healthcare models.

In 1990, one of Dr. Ornish's most well-known research revealed, for the first time, that individuals with heart disease might repair coronary artery blockages by thorough lifestyle modifications. Following Dr. Ornish's approach resulted in significant improvements in cardiac function, decreased chest pain, and the reversal of coronary artery blockages after just one year, according to the Lifestyle Heart Trial study.

Numerous accolades, such as the Smithsonian American Ingenuity Award in Health and Medicine, the Bravewell Collaborative Pioneer of Integrative Medicine Award, and the esteemed University of Texas at Austin Outstanding Young Alumnus Award, have been bestowed upon Dr. Ornish in recognition of his widely acknowledged body of work.

Dr. Ornish has published multiple best-selling books, including "Dr. Dean Ornish's Program for Reversing Heart Disease," "Eat More, Weigh

Less," and "The Spectrum." In addition to his research, Dr. Ornish has held positions as a clinical professor of medicine at the University of California, San Francisco and as a member of the American Heart Association's board of directors.

Dr. Dean Ornish has changed our understanding of the connection between lifestyle and health through his writings, research, and advocacy work. He has motivated millions of people worldwide to adopt healthier lifestyles and prevent and reverse chronic diseases through social support, exercise, diet, and stress management.

The foundation of Dr. Dean Ornish's Ornish Program for Reversing Heart Disease is comprised of four essential pillars, which are referred to as the "Four Pillars of Health." These pillars signify the primary areas of emphasis for reaching the highest possible level of health and wellness. Among them are:

Healthy Eating: The Ornish Program's first pillar highlights the value of a plant-based, whole-foods-based diet that is minimal in processed foods, fat, and refined carbs. A range of fruits, vegetables, whole grains, legumes, and plant-based proteins should be consumed by participants, but consumption of animal products, added sweets, and harmful fats should be kept to a minimum. The diet's abundance in fiber, vitamins, minerals, and antioxidants can help lower cholesterol, lessen inflammation, and enhance heart health.

Frequent Exercise: The Ornish Program's second pillar highlights the importance of regular exercise in fostering cardiovascular health and general well-being. On most days of the week, participants are urged to perform moderate-intensity aerobic exercise for at least 30 minutes, such as brisk walking or cycling. To increase muscle strength and endurance, strength training activities like lifting weights or utilizing resistance bands are advised to be done at least twice a week.

CHAPTER TWO

Stress Management: In order to support mental and emotional well-being, stress reduction strategies are the third pillar of the Ornish Program. The program incorporates several stress management strategies, including deep breathing exercises, yoga, mindfulness, and meditation. By lowering stress, worry, and negative emotions, these techniques assist people in improving their mental and physical health.

Social Support: The Ornish Program's fourth pillar highlights the value of social support and relationships in fostering health and wellbeing. Strong social bonds have been linked to longer lifespans and improved health outcomes, according to research. Building and sustaining supportive relationships with family, friends, and community members is encouraged by the curriculum. Online forums, instructional courses, and group support sessions are frequently offered to encourage a sense of accountability and connection among members.

Heart disease and other chronic illnesses can be prevented and reversed with the help of the Ornish Program, which focuses on four key areas: stress management, social support, regular exercise, and balanced diet. Through learning how to modify their lifestyle in a sustainable way, participants can enhance their quality of life and long-term vitality while also supporting their health and well-being.

Advantages of the Ornish Program for Health

Decades of scientific research and clinical data support the many health benefits of the Ornish Program for Reversing Heart Disease. The following are some of the main health advantages of the Ornish Program:

Better Heart Health: Preventing and treating heart disease is one of the main objectives of the Ornish Program. Studies have indicated that those who adhere to the regimen see notable improvements in their cardiovascular health, including lower blood pressure, cholesterol, and arterial plaque accumulation. A decreased risk of heart attacks, strokes, and other cardiovascular events may result from these advancements.

Weight Management: The Ornish Program is a useful strategy for managing weight because it places an emphasis on a whole-foods-based, plant-based diet that is low in fat and processed carbs. Weight loss or maintenance is common among participants, and it can lower the chance of developing obesity-related diseases such type 2 diabetes, hypertension, and metabolic syndrome.

Reduced Inflammation: Heart disease, diabetes, cancer, and autoimmune disorders are just a few of the chronic diseases that are associated to systemic inflammation, which can be lessened by following the Ornish Program's plant-based diet, which has anti-inflammatory properties. The program may help lower the risk of chronic disease and enhance general health by lowering inflammation.

Better Blood Sugar Control: People with prediabetes, type 2 diabetes, or insulin resistance may benefit from the Ornish Program's emphasis on whole, unprocessed foods and low-glycemic carbs, which can help stabilize blood sugar levels and increase insulin sensitivity.

Improved Mental Well-Being: An essential part of the Ornish Program, stress-reduction methods like yoga, mindfulness, and meditation can help lower levels of stress, anxiety, and depression. Practicing these stress-reduction tactics is associated with higher mood, increased emotional resilience, and enhanced general well-being, according to participant reports.

Enhanced Energy and Vitality: Eating a plant-based, whole-food diet and exercising on a regular basis can increase energy levels, improve the quality of sleep, and improve general vitality. As participants integrate the Ornish Program's principals into their lifestyle, they frequently report feeling more energised, getting better sleep, and being more resilient to fatigue.

Improved Quality of Life: The Ornish Program can improve participants' quality of life by addressing several aspects of well-being and encouraging holistic health. Making lasting lifestyle adjustments that promote lifespan and health has been associated with increased vibrancy, engagement, and fulfillment, according to numerous reports.

All things considered, the Ornish Program provides a thorough approach to health and wellness that tackles the root causes of chronic illness and gives people the tools they need to take charge of their health via nutrition, exercise, stress reduction, and social support. Adopting the Ornish Program's tenets can help people enhance their general quality of life and reap a host of health advantages.

Accepting an Ornish Way of Life

To achieve optimal health and well-being, adopting the Ornish lifestyle entails making significant adjustments to your food, exercise regimen, stress-reduction techniques, and social network. To assist you in making the switch to the Ornish lifestyle, here are some steps:

Become Informed: Invest some time in learning about the fundamentals of the Ornish way of life, such as the significance of a plant-based, whole-food diet, frequent exercise, stress reduction methods, and social support. Learn about the scientific proof that certain lifestyle modifications are beneficial in avoiding and treating chronic illnesses.

Transition to a Plant-Based Diet: Reduce your intake of animal products, added sugars, and harmful fats by gradually switching to a plant-based diet that places an emphasis on fruits, vegetables, whole grains, legumes, and plant-based proteins. Try out new recipes, look at plant-based substitutes for dairy and meat, and come up with inventive methods to include more plant-based foods in your meals.

Include Regular Exercise: Include moderate-intensity aerobic exercise for at least 30 minutes on most days of the week to include physical activity into your routine. To increase muscle strength and endurance, incorporate enjoyable activities like walking, cycling, swimming, or dancing. You should also try to incorporate strength training exercises at least twice a week.

Practice Stress Management Techniques: To assist lower stress, anxiety, and negative emotions, incorporate stress management techniques like deep breathing exercises, yoga, mindfulness, meditation, and tai chi into your daily routine. Prioritize the practices that you find meaningful for your mental and emotional health.

Cultivate Social Connections: To encourage social interaction and emotional support, cultivate ties of support with neighbors, family, and friends. Engage in online forums, instructional courses, or support groups to meet people who have similar health objectives and experiences.

Establish Achievable and objective Goals: Divide your adoption of the Ornish lifestyle into smaller, more doable steps by setting attainable and objective goals. Pay attention to the small adjustments you make over time, and acknowledge your accomplishments as you go. It takes time and effort to embrace a new lifestyle, so be patient with yourself.

Seek Accountability and Support: Be in the company of people who will motivate and inspire you to stick with your health-related objectives. For extra support and accountability, think about joining a support group, getting in touch with friends and family, or hiring a health coach or certified nutritionist.

Remain Open-Minded and Flexible: As you traverse the Ornish lifestyle, welcome experimentation and adaptability. Try a variety of foods, pastimes, and stress-reduction strategies; pay attention to your body's signals to figure out what suits you best. Continue to be inquisitive, involved, and dedicated to your path to the best possible health and wellbeing.

You can reap many health benefits and enhance your general quality of life by embracing the Ornish lifestyle and implementing its tenets into your everyday activities. Always keep in mind that little adjustments over time can have a large impact and that any action you take to improve your health is a positive one.

Meal Ideas and Recipes That Are Ornish-Friendly

Adopting an Ornish-friendly diet entails consuming as few animal products, added sugars, and harmful fats as possible while emphasizing entire, plant-based foods. To get you started, check out these tasty and wholesome Ornish-friendly recipes and meal ideas:

Vegetable Stir-Fry: In a small quantity of vegetable broth or water, sauté a variety of vibrant veggies, including bell peppers, broccoli, carrots, snap peas, and mushrooms. Add ginger and garlic as well as tamari or low-sodium soy sauce for seasoning. For a filling supper, serve over quinoa or brown rice.

In a bowl, mix cooked black beans, corn kernels, diced tomatoes, chopped red onion, and chopped cilantro for the Black Bean and Corn Salad. Mix together lime juice, olive oil, chile powder, cumin, and minced garlic to dress. Serve as a cool salad or as a whole-grain tortilla filler.

Mushroom and Spinach Frittata: In a nonstick skillet, cook diced onions, chopped spinach, and sliced mushrooms until soft. Add a splash of unsweetened almond milk and whisk together eggs or egg substitute in a separate bowl. Season with salt, pepper, and herbs. Cover the veggies with the egg mixture and simmer until it sets. Serve this as a wholesome breakfast or brunch option with a side of mixed greens.

Lentil Soup: Cook chopped carrots, celery, onions, and garlic in vegetable stock with dried lentils until the lentils are soft. Use seasonings like as paprika, cumin, bay leaves, and thyme. For a cozy and filling supper, top with a sliver of whole-grain bread and garnish with fresh parsley.

Marinate portobello mushroom caps in a mixture of garlic, olive oil, balsamic vinegar, and herbs for at least half an hour before grilling. For a simple yet delectable entrée, grill or roast the mushrooms until they are soft. Serve with a side of steamed vegetables or a mixed green salad.

Tofu Veggie Stir-Fry: A tasty sauce consisting of low-sodium soy sauce, garlic, ginger, and a hint of maple syrup or agave nectar is stir-fried with cubed tofu and a variety of veggies, including bell peppers, broccoli, snow peas, and carrots. Serve over whole-grain noodles or brown rice for a filling, high-protein supper.

Sandwich with Chickpea Salad: Mash cooked chickpeas with avocado, lemon juice, chopped celery, red onion, and parsley or cilantro, as well as minced garlic. For more taste, season with salt, pepper, and a small teaspoon of cayenne. For a tasty and substantial sandwich, spread the chickpea salad across whole-grain bread or lettuce leaves.

Roasted Vegetable Medley: Combine chopped veggies with herbs, garlic, and olive oil, including sweet potatoes, Brussels sprouts, cauliflower, and red onions. Roast in the oven until caramelized and brown. To make it a full meal, top with cooked nutritious grains like farro or quinoa and serve as a side dish.

In addition to being scrumptious and filling, these Ornish-friendly dishes and meal ideas are also nutrient-rich, supporting your general health and wellbeing. You are welcome to alter them to suit your dietary requirements and preferences. Enjoy discovering the variety of tastes and sensations that come with a plant-based diet!

Advice for Social Events and Eating Out

Following the Ornish lifestyle while navigating social events and eating out might be doable with enough preparation and awareness. When dining out or attending social events, the following advice will help you make better decisions and maintain your discipline:

Examine Menus in Advance: Spend some time online reviewing the menu before going out to eat. Seek out eateries that provide plant-based selections or recipes that are easily adaptable to your dietary requirements. These days, a lot of eaties include vegan or vegetarian options; some even mark their food as low-fat or heart-healthy.

Pick Wisely: Go for eateries that put an emphasis on using whole, fresh products and providing a variety of customizable options. Plant-based foods from various ethnic cuisines, including Mediterranean, Asian, and Mexican, are a good fit for the Ornish way of life. Steer clear of fast food chains and eateries that specialize in processed, high-fat menu items.

Emphasis on Plant-Based Options: When looking through the menu, give special attention to plant-based foods that include fruits, vegetables, whole grains, legumes, and nuts. Scan for salads, bean-based dishes, stir-fries, grain bowls, grilled or roasted vegetable platters, and soups made with vegetables. To reduce extra sugar and fat and to limit portion sizes, ask for dressings, sauces, and garnishes on the side.

Ask for Modifications: Don't be afraid to ask your server to make changes to accommodate your dietary requirements. Ask for sauces or dressings to be provided on the side and request that dishes be cooked with as little oil, butter, or cheese added as possible. Special requests are usually accommodated by restaurants, particularly if they are made for health-related reasons.

Be Aware of Portions: When dining out, be mindful of the portion sizes since restaurant dishes are frequently greater than what you would normally eat at home. In order to cut down on the quantity of food offered, think about splitting an entree with a dining partner or requesting a half portion. As an alternative, divide your meal in half and store it for later.

Watch What You Drink: Sugary sodas, sweetened teas, and alcoholic drinks are examples of high-calorie drinks that should be avoided as they can lead to overindulgence in calories. Instead, go for unsweetened beverages, herbal teas, sparkling water with lime or lemon, or water. If you decide to use alcohol, use it sparingly and think about healthier options like wine or spritzers.

Exercise Moderation: It's acceptable to periodically indulge in addition to making healthy decisions. Allow yourself to indulge guilt-free in a little quantity of your favorite food or dessert if you're celebrating or dining out. Without overindulging, concentrate on experiencing the flavors and the occasion.

Plan Ahead for Social Events: To assist stifle hunger and avoid overindulging, if you're going a social event or gathering where food will be offered, think about having a small, nutrient-rich meal or snack beforehand. In order to ensure that there are healthy options accessible, offer to bring one or two dishes that fit the Ornish lifestyle.

Remember that social gatherings are about more than just the food; instead, concentrate on enjoying the company. Put your attention on spending time with friends and family, having deep discussions, and doing things that make you happy. Turn your attention from eating to the relationships and experiences that are really important.

You may confidently negotiate eating out and social gatherings while adhering to your Ornish lifestyle goals if you put these guidelines into practice. You may maintain your health and well-being while still enjoying delectable meals and fulfilling social interactions with a little preparation and awareness.

Practicing mindfulness and stress-reduction methods on a regular basis can assist your Ornish lifestyle objectives and enhance your general well-being. The following useful advice will help you incorporate stress-reduction and mindfulness techniques into your daily routine:

Start Each Day Mindfully: Take a few minutes to practice mindful breathing or meditation at the start of each day. Shut your eyes, take a few deep breaths, and concentrate on how your breath feels entering and exiting your body. Make a grateful list for the current moment and set a good purpose for the day.

Practice Mindful Eating: During meals and snacks, be aware of your eating habits and engage in mindful eating. Savor every bite of your food by chewing it carefully and focusing on its flavor, texture, and scent. Steer clear of electronics like TVs, phones, and laptops, and whenever you can, try to dine in a peaceful, quiet setting.

Take Brief Mindfulness Breaks: Throughout the day, make time to practice mindfulness and focus on the here and now by taking brief breaks. Take a few minutes to check in with your physical and mental well-being, pay attention to your breathing, or simply study your surroundings. These brief moments of awareness can aid in lowering tension and promoting emotions of serenity and relaxation.

Include Movement-Based Mindfulness: To assist lower stress and encourage relaxation, try movement-based mindfulness exercises like yoga, tai chi, or qigong. These easy, flowing movements enhance flexibility, balance, and general well-being by fusing conscious movement with breath awareness.

Develop a Daily Gratitude Practice: Set aside some time each day to consider the things for which you are thankful. No matter how big or little, list three things every day for which you are grateful in a gratitude diary. You can change your viewpoint and cultivate positive and content feelings by concentrating on your thankfulness.

Establish Technology Boundaries: Restrict your time spent on screens and digital gadgets, especially before bed. Establish limits on the amount of time you spend using technology and designate areas of your house like the dining room or bedroom that are free of electronics. Throughout the day, take regular breaks from screens to prevent eye strain and brain exhaustion.

Practice Relaxation Techniques: To help you decompress and unwind, try incorporating progressive muscle relaxation, guided imagery, or body scans into your everyday routine. Try out a variety of methods to see which one suits you the most, and then practice frequently to get the most out of it.

Connect with Nature: Spend as much time as you can outside in the great outdoors, since it has a calming effect on both the body and the mind. Go for a stroll in the park, a ramble through the forest, or just sit outside and enjoy the sights and sounds of nature. Making a connection with nature can improve mood, lower stress levels, and general wellbeing.

Seek Connection and Support: If you're looking for emotional support and connection, get in touch with friends, family, or support groups. Talk about your feelings, ideas, and experiences with people who can relate to and validate your path. Creating a strong support system can help foster a sense of community and belonging while easing stress and feelings of loneliness.

CHAPTER THREE

You can support your Ornish lifestyle objectives and build a deeper sense of calm, resilience, and well-being by implementing these mindfulness and stress reduction methods into your daily life. To reap the full advantages of mindfulness and stress reduction in your life, start small and build upon your practice gradually over time.

Sustaining Drive and Advancement

Long-term success on your Ornish lifestyle path requires you to stay motivated and make progress. The following tactics will support your motivation and enable you to keep moving forward with your wellness and health goals:

Set Achievable, Specific, Measurable, and practical Goals: Make sure your goals are practical, measurable, and well-defined. Divide more ambitious objectives into more doable benchmarks, and acknowledge your advancements as you go. To maintain your goals challenging and relevant, evaluate them frequently and make any adjustments.

Discover Your Why: Determine the specific reasons you choose to live an Ornish lifestyle, and keep these reasons close to your heart on a frequent basis. Reaching out to your underlying motivations can help you stay committed and goal-focused, whether your focus is on heart health, weight loss, energy, or just feeling better all around.

Emphasize Progress Rather than Perfection: Accept the path of ongoing development and place more emphasis on progress than perfection. Acknowledge that obstacles and disappointments are an inherent aspect of any lifestyle transition and see them as chances for development. Throughout your wellness journey, remember to treat yourself with kindness and self-compassion.

Honor Your Accomplishments: Honor your accomplishments, no matter how modest, and give credit for your perseverance and hard work along the way. When you hit significant milestones, treat yourself to incentives or rewards. Some examples of these are a well-deserved spa day, a brand-new fitness equipment, or a nutritious dinner at your preferred eatery.

Remain Consistent: Seeing outcomes over time and keeping momentum require consistency. Create daily routines and behaviors that help you achieve your Ornish lifestyle objectives, such as eating balanced meals, exercising, managing your stress, and placing self-care first. Make a constant effort to eat healthily, especially on days when you're not feeling very motivated.

Find Accountability and Support: Be in the company of friends, family, or other Ornish participants who are understanding and encouraging of your path. To help you keep motivated and on track, find accountability partners or support groups. You can also share your objectives and struggles with others.

Track Your Progress: Keep tabs on important indicators like weight, blood pressure, cholesterol, physical activity, and stress levels to be informed about your progress. Keep a notebook, logbook, or tracker to document your daily routine, successes, and setbacks. Review your progress often to spot patterns, acknowledge triumphs, and make modifications as needed.

Stay Educated and Informed: Stay informed on the newest research, resources, and advances relevant to the Ornish lifestyle and overall health and wellness. Attend workshops, webinars, or support group meetings to learn new tactics, share experiences, and connect with others who share your goals.

Visualize Success: Visualize yourself attaining your goals and enjoying your best life as a result of your efforts. Create vision boards, affirmations, or mental visualization exercises to help you stay focused, motivated, and inspired. Visualizing success can help strengthen your dedication and keep you pushing forward, especially when faced with setbacks.

Be Flexible and Adapt: Be willing to adapt and change your strategy as needed to overcome difficulties and stay on track toward your goals. Remain open to attempting new ideas, experimenting with different techniques, and seeking alternate answers when faced with setbacks or impediments. Remember that flexibility and resilience are crucial to long-term success.

By implementing these tactics into your daily routine, you can maintain motivation, stay on track with your Ornish lifestyle objectives, and continue making progress toward greater health and well-being. Remember that change takes time and patience, so be gentle with yourself and stay devoted to your journey of self-improvement and growth.

Testimonials and Success Stories

Success stories and testimonies from individuals who have embraced the Ornish lifestyle can be motivating and motivational for those considering or already on a similar journey. Here are a few examples of success stories and testimonials from individuals who have achieved excellent effects with the Ornish lifestyle:

Reversal of Heart Disease: "I was resolved to take charge of my health and stay away from intrusive surgeries after receiving a heart disease diagnosis. I gained knowledge about how to handle stress, switch to a plant-based diet, and fit regular exercise into my schedule thanks to the Ornish Program. My blood pressure returned to normal, my cholesterol levels decreased, and I was able to stop taking medication in a matter of months. I've been able to reverse my cardiac disease and restore my vitality and quality of life because of the Ornish lifestyle."

Weight Loss and Energy Boost: "Knowing I had to change, I was struggling with extra weight and lack energy. I read about the health benefits of the Ornish lifestyle and made the decision to give it a try. I gained much more energy and vitality in addition to losing weight by switching to a plant-based diet and implementing mindfulness exercises into my daily routine. I feel better than ever lighter, more alive, and more assured. My life has been completely changed by the Ornish lifestyle."

Better Control of Diabetes: "Despite taking medicine and following dietary guidelines, I found it difficult to control my blood sugar levels for years after being diagnosed with type 2 diabetes. Upon learning about the Ornish

Program, I was hesitant at first but decided to give it a shot. To my surprise, my blood sugar levels started to stabilize and I was able to cut back on my medication dosage a few weeks after switching to a plant-based diet and exercising stress-reduction tactics. I'm happier and healthier than ever now because of the Ornish way of life."

Enhanced Emotional Well-Being: "I felt like I was trapped in a loop of negativity and despair since I was dealing with chronic stress, anxiety, and depression. I looked to the Ornish way of life for solace and direction. I developed stress management, mental quietness, and inner calm through self-care, mindfulness, and meditation techniques. My anxiety has decreased, my mood has improved, and I feel more centered and balanced in my day-to-day activities as a result. For me, the Ornish way of life has been indispensable."

These testimonials and success stories demonstrate how the Ornish lifestyle can improve overall health, wellbeing, and quality of life. People's physical, emotional, and mental health can significantly improve by adopting a plant-based diet, exercising frequently, learning stress management techniques, and building supportive relationships. These tales serve as powerful reminders of the potential advantages and favorable results that await you on your personal path to optimum health and wellness if you're thinking about adopting the Ornish lifestyle.

CONCLUSION

To sum up, the Ornish way of life emphasizes nurturing the body, mind, and spirit in order to promote overall health and wholeness. A plant-based diet, consistent exercise, stress-reduction techniques, and building supportive relationships can all help people achieve significant improvements in their overall health, wellbeing, and quality of life.

We have personally witnessed the transformative impact of the Ornish lifestyle via the success stories and testimonials of those who have adopted it. These include managing weight, improving mental well-being, controlling diabetes, and reversing heart disease. These incredible testimonies attest to the Ornish lifestyle's effectiveness in enhancing long-term health and vitality.

As you set out on your personal path to optimal health and well-being, keep in mind that transformation requires persistence, patience, and commitment. Treat yourself well, recognize your accomplishments, and remain committed to your objectives. Whether your goal is to manage chronic illnesses, strengthen your heart, or just feel better overall, the Ornish lifestyle provides a comprehensive framework for achieving long-term results.

Through the incorporation of Ornish living principles into your everyday routine and long-lasting lifestyle modifications, you can reap the profound advantages of a plant-based diet, consistent exercise, stress reduction, and social support. Accept the journey, maintain your motivation, and have faith in your ability to improve your health and change your life.

THE END

www.ingramcontent.com/pod-product-compliance
Lightning Source LLC
Chambersburg PA
CBHW051920250726

48659CB00002B/745